How This Book Is Set Up

✓ **Find out exactly what plantar fasciitis is in** *Chapter 1*.

✓ **Understand the typical course of plantar fasciitis in** *Chapter 2*.

✓ **Learn the** *5-Minute Plantar Fasciitis Solution* **in** *Chapter 3*.

✓ **Monitor your progress every few weeks with the tools in** *Chapter 4*.

✓ **Discover what you can do to prevent it from coming back in** *Chapter 5*.

Why Is The Print In This Book So Big?

People who read my books sometimes wonder why the print is so big in many of them. Some tend to think it's because I'm trying to make a little book bigger or a short book longer.

Actually, the main reason I use bigger print is for the same reason I intentionally write short books, usually under 100 pages–it's just plain easier to read and get the information quicker!

You see, the books I write address common, everyday problems that people of *all* ages have. In other words, the "typical" reader of my books could be a teenager, a busy housewife, a CEO, a construction worker, or a retired senior citizen with poor eyesight. Therefore, by writing books with larger print that are short and to the point, *everyone* can get the information quickly and with ease. After all, what good is a book full of useful information if nobody ever finishes it?

The 5-Minute Plantar Fasciitis Solution

by
Jim Johnson, PT

Drawings and Cover Art by Eunice Johnson
Cover Design by Christa and Tim Johnson

This edition published by
Dog Ear Publishing
4010 W. 86th Street, Ste H
Indianapolis, IN 46268

www.dogearpublishing.net

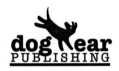

ISBN: 978-159858-551-3
Library of Congress Control Number:
This book is printed on acid-free paper.

Printed in the United States of America

Table of Contents

I have given my best effort to ensure that this book is entirely based upon scientific evidence and not on intuition, single case reports, opinions of authorities, anecdotal evidence, or unsystematic clinical observations. Where I do express my opinion in this book, it is directly stated as such.

—*Jim Johnson, P.T.*

Chapter One

What The Heck Is *Plantar Fasciitis*?

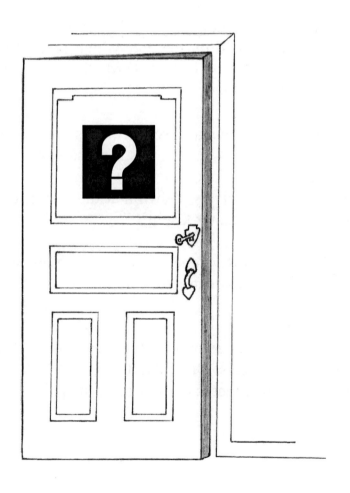

What The Heck Is *Plantar Fasciitis*?

If you're like a lot of my patients, you probably have trouble even saying the words "plantar fasciitis"– I know I did when I came across them in physical therapy school. So, let's start there.

Plantar fasciitis is commonly pronounced *plan-tar fash-eye-tiss*. Breaking it down, the word *plantar* refers to the sole of the foot. *Fasciitis*, on the other hand, is a combination of the word "fascia" (Latin for band), with the suffix "itis" tacked on the end–which refers to inflammation. Put 'em all together, and you've got two words that mean inflammation of the bands on the sole of your foot.

But while this is what plantar fasciitis means *literally*, a careful review of the published research shows us that this is actually not a good description at all of what is going on. Nope, the plain truth of the matter is that many, many studies have conclusively shown that there is in fact *no* inflammation involved when one has "plantar fasciitis."

Surprised? You're not alone. Confused? You won't be for long. Skeptical? Well, I consider that a good thing.

In the pages that follow, I'll explain exactly what this annoying condition is, what you can do about it, and back up everything I say with published research and clinical studies. So without any further delay, let's take a close look at the very structure that is the source of the pain, *the plantar fascia…*

The Plantar Fascia

The plantar fascia, is a broad band of fibrous tissue that runs along the bottom of your foot. It starts out from your heel area and then begins to "fan out" as it heads towards each of your individual toes. Here's a closer look:

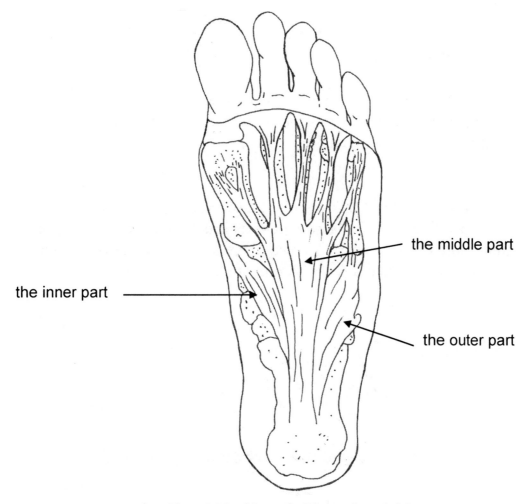

the middle part

the inner part

the outer part

Figure 1.1 Looking at the bottom of your left foot– the three major parts of the plantar fascia.

As you can see, the plantar fascia can be divided up into three major areas: an inner, outer, and middle part. However it is only the *middle* part that we're mainly concerned with in this book. This is for several reasons:

- the inner and outer parts of the plantar fascia are not nearly as important to the functioning of your foot as the middle part.

- the inner part is a really thin structure that mainly serves to cover other foot structures.

- the outer part serves to cover other foot structures as well, and its development can vary quite a lot. In fact, it is virtually *absent* in about 7% of people (Hedrick 1996).

So from now on, when I talk about "the plantar fascia" in this book, I'll be referring specifically to the *middle* part, as it is by far the most important of the three (more on that later). Anyway, here are some more basic pictures to give you a look at it from a few different angles:

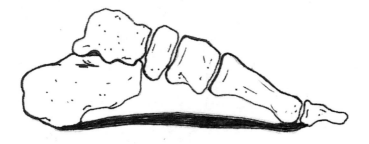

Figure 1.2 Looking at the plantar fascia from the side.

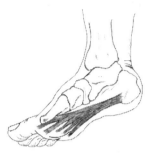

Figure 1.3 A bottom view of the plantar fascia.

So What Exactly Is Fascia Anyway?

Well, fascia is a type of connective tissue that can be found just about everywhere in your body, not just in your foot. Made up of *collagen* and *elastin* fibers, there's a layer of this fascia stuff right under your skin, around your organs, and for that matter, even around each of your muscles! Best thought of as a kind of "packing material," one of the big jobs of fascia is to provide support to the many different structures throughout your body.

Not all fascia is created equal however. For example, some of the fascia in your body is laid out much like a thin sheet of tissue paper. If you've ever removed the skin from a chicken breast, that white film-like substance right underneath the skin you may have noticed was actually a very thin layer of fascia–which is quite similar to how it looks in humans too.

The *plantar* fascia in your foot, on the other hand, is not nearly this thin. Just how thin is it? Well, I looked into this matter one time and quickly realized that while many studies were so nicely reporting the thickness of the plantar fascia, each researcher seemed to be measuring it from a different spot on the bottom of your foot! So, the only way to really get to the "bottom" of things was to group these studies based upon the location where they were measuring the plantar fascia, and then write down all the numbers. The following page is the result of one of my more tedious literature searches, but the work was well worth it and I was finally able to sort things out. As you can see with a quick scan of the tables, your normal plantar fascia is somewhere around 3 mm (millimeters) thick. However when you have plantar fasciitis, the fascia actually gets *thicker*, reaching around the 5 to 6 millimeter range–or more!

Studies That Have Measured the Plantar Fascia

Studies where the plantar fascia was measured exactly 5 mm from its attachment to the heel bone.

study	average thickness in plantar fasciitis patients	average thickness in normal/control group	technique used
Uzel 2006	-	3.1 mm	ultrasound
Ozdemir 2005	2.9 mm	2.5 mm	ultrasound
Wall 1993	5.6 mm	3.5 mm	ultrasound

Studies where the plantar fascia was measured at some point within 5 cm from its attachment to the heel bone.

study	average thickness in plantar fasciitis patients	average thickness in normal/control group	technique used
Osborne 2006	5.6 mm	3.2 mm	X-ray
Uzel 2006	-	3.6 mm	ultrasound
Zhu 2005	6 to 7 mm	-	MRI
Giacomozzi 2005	-	2.0 mm	ultrasound
Akfirat 2003	4.7 mm	3.6 mm	ultrasound
Berkowitz 1991	7.4 mm	3.2 mm	MRI

Studies where the plantar fascia was measured at the point where it crosses under the front edge of your heel bone.

study	average thickness in plantar fasciitis patients	average thickness in normal/control group	technique used
Sabir 2005	5.6 mm	3.0 mm	MRI
Sabir 2005	4.9 mm	3.2 mm	ultrasound
Genc 2005	6.2 mm	3.5 mm	ultrasound
Kane 2001	5.7 mm	3.8 mm	ultrasound
Kamel 2000	5.8 mm	2.4 mm	ultrasound
Gibbon 1999	6.0 mm	3.3 mm	ultrasound

What Does the Plantar Fascia Do?

While the plantar fascia serves many different purposes, such as helping to protect the underside of your foot, by far its most commonly cited function in the scientific literature is its critical role in *supporting the arch of your foot*. Here's a basic picture of the plantar fascia and a foot arch to show you just how closely the two are related:

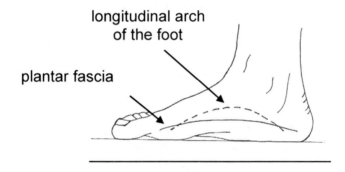

Figure 1.4 Looking at the right foot from the side– the plantar fascia and the arch of your foot that it supports.

As you can see, you have the arch of your foot, with the plantar fascia running along its entire base (Figure 1.4). Now since the plantar fascia connects at *both* ends of your foot arch, it is in the perfect position to act as a kind of "tie-rod" to help stabilize the arch under the weight of your body. Here's a few of the many studies that have confirmed this arch supporting function of the plantar fascia:

- a study done on cadavers (bodies donated to science) found that when the plantar fascia was completely cut and released, the foot arch dropped severely (Murphy 1998).

- another cadaver study calculated that after the plantar fascia was completely cut, arch stiffness decreased by twenty-five percent (Huang 1993).

Now that you know how the plantar fascia supports the arch of your foot while you're standing, let's discuss how the plantar fascia supports it while you're walking. Mechanically speaking, it's through a way known as *the windlass mechanism*. Let me explain.

A windlass is simply a certain kind of of hauling or lifting device you've probably seen at one time or another but didn't know it had a fancy name. It's made up of some cable or rope which is wound around a cylinder. The cylinder is then turned by a crank or motor, and when this happens–presto, up comes the load. Here's a picture of your basic windlass:

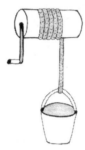

Figure 1.5 The windlass.

Now believe it or not, the plantar fascia works this very same way to support your foot arch as you're walking. Here's how:

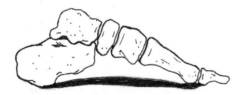
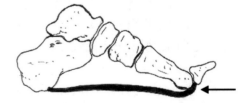

Figure 1.6 Side view of the plantar fascia when your foot is at rest. Note that the plantar fascia goes all the way up to your toes.

Figure 1.7 Now look what happens when the toes are raised– the arch is higher! Raising the toes up has wound the plantar fascia around the foot bones (arrow) which pulls the fascia tighter and in turn helps raise the arch. This action is called *the windlass mechanism*.

So just as the rope gets wound tight around the cylinder in the windlass device as the crank is turned (Figure 1.5), so is the plantar fascia wound tighter around your foot bones as the toes are raised. And when this happens, the plantar fascia helps out to raise your foot arch up and make it _super-stable_ when you need it the most–like when you're walking or climbing stairs. Figure 1.8 shows us what the windlass mechanism looks like in action _each time we take a step_:

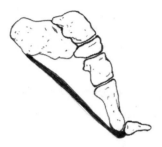

Figure 1.8 The windlass mechanism goes into action every time you take a step. With the toes bent up, the plantar fascia becomes tighter and helps raise up the arch– which makes it more stable as you put all your weight on one foot while walking.

Know too that there has been much research conducted over the years which has confirmed that these things actually take place. For instance, many studies have shown that:

- the foot arch does indeed rise as the toes are bent (Hicks 1954, Kappel-Bargas 1998)

  and

- the foot arch rises from step to step as we walk (Cashmere 1999, Hunt 2001).

So as you can see, because of its attachments from one end of the foot to the other, the plantar fascia is working hard to support our foot arches against the weight of our body all day long–not only when we're simply standing still on our feet, but also through the windlass mechanism as we're walking around.

Doesn't the plantar fascia get inflammed?

There was a time when I thought so too–until I did a thorough literature search and found out otherwise. There are several reasons for this popular misconception and a big one has to do with the way people are typically diagnosed with plantar fasciitis. For instance, most people are commonly told that they have plantar fasciitis based on several things:

- the symptoms they are having (i.e. heel pain, especially with the first few steps in the morning or after a period of inactivity)

- the results of their physical exam (i.e. pain on the bottom of the foot when pressed on, most often in the heel area)

- nothing else obvious is going on (i.e. no broken bones, not related to a disease a person may have)

As you can see, we really have no nifty little X-ray or lab tests doctors can run that will tell them that a patient definitely has plantar fasciitis. Furthermore, none of the above things that are commonly used to diagnosis plantar fasciitis are really proof positive that there is indeed inflammation present in the fascia. And so, since we don't have any definitive tests for plantar fasciitis, people who are told they have this condition automatically assume that their fascia is chock-full of inflammation. But is this *really* the case?

Well, if we approach this matter scientifically, to say that something is "inflammed" means that we should be able to find some hard evidence of inflammation. Now without getting too caught up in details, inflammation can be broken down into two general patterns, *acute* and *chronic*.

Here's the difference between the two:

- *acute inflammation* is an immediate and early response to tissue injury. It comes on quick, but lasts for minutes, hours, or a few days. Neutrophils are the major kind of cells that are involved in acute inflammation.

- *chronic inflammation* is inflammation of a prolonged duration, such as weeks or months, in which active inflammation, tissue destruction, and repair are all going on at the same time. Some of the major types of cells that are involved in chronic inflammation include macrophages, lymphocytes, and plasma cells.

It's not important to know all about the different types of cells, although you may be interested to know that a lot of them are simply different types of white blood cells. What is important, however, is to know that these are exactly the kinds of cells we should be able to find in people with plantar fasciitis *if* the fascia is indeed "inflammed"–since these are the cells directly involved in the body's inflammatory process. So now that you have this knowledge, let's see what researchers have found:

study	# of samples	average duration of symptoms	major histological findings reported
Lemont 2003	**50**	**"chronic"**	**-myxoid degeneration with fragmentation and degeneration of the plantar fsscia**
Jarde 2003	**38**	**2 yrs.**	**-cartilaginous metaplasia, chondroid or osteoid metaplasia, fibromatosis, microcalcifications**
Tountas 1996	**21**	**10.6 months**	**-mucoid and fibrinoid degeneration of plantar fascia**
Leach 1986	**16**	**7 months to 2 yrs**	**-chronic granulomatous tissue -mucinoid degeneration**
Snider 1983	**10**	**20.5 months**	**-collagen degeneration, chondroid metaplasia, angiofibroblastic hyperplasia, matrix calcification**

What this table represents is the result of a literature search I did one time when I was looking for *all* the studies that took at least ten people diagnosed with plantar fasciitis, removed a piece of their fascia, and looked at it under a microscope. And, as you can see, it doesn't look like researchers have reported finding many of the cells that are directly involved in the inflammatory process. Therefore, without some cellular proof of an inflammatory response, one has no basis to accurately say that the plantar fascia is indeed "inflammed" when one has plantar fasciitis.

> ***The point:*** Inflammation does *not* appear to be a major feature of plantar fasciitis, especially in patients that have been suffering with this condition for many months. Studies do, however, *consistently* find evidence of degenerative changes in the fascia.

This is probably the single most important piece of information to know when it comes to unlocking the mystery of getting rid of plantar fasciitis. Realizing that the main problem is actually one of *failed healing*, not inflammation, means that a successful treatment *must* be one that creates a healing environment for the plantar fascia to finally repair itself.

Summary

✓ the plantar fascia is a broad band of fibrous tissue that runs along the bottom of your foot, going from your heel all the way to your toes

✓ plantar fascia is a type of connective tissue made up of collagen and elastin fibers

✓ a big job of the plantar fascia is to support the arch of your foot while you're standing and walking

✓ while you are walking, the plantar fascia supports your foot arch through *the windlass mechanism*

✓ studies that have taken people with plantar fasciitis and examined their fascia under a microscope consistently find degenerative changes in the fascia, *not* inflammation

Chapter Two

How Long Does Plantar Fasciitis Last?

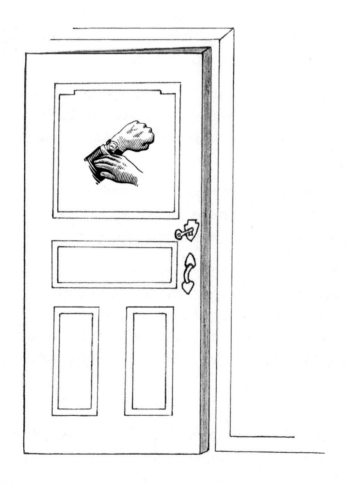

How Long Does Plantar Fasciitis Last?

It's on the mind of everyone who has it. Scientifically speaking, the only way to know for sure how long plantar fasciitis typically lasts, is to conduct what is called a *natural history study*. Natural history studies attempt to find out exactly how long a disease (or problem) will last on its own, naturally, without interference, by following a group of patients over time that receive *no medical treatment*. Problem is, while there are natural history studies for many different medical conditions, none have been done on plantar fasciitis. Apparently, people suffering with plantar fasciitis are hesitant to skip medical treatment for the sake of science!

But before you get *too* discouraged, let me tell you what you will find when sifting through the research–studies on the typical course of plantar fasciitis *when managed non-operatively* (without surgery). The studies go something like this:

- researchers gather records of people who have had plantar fasciitis
- they find out when the symptoms started and when they resolved
- they find out exactly what treatments they got

While you won't be able to figure out the *true* natural course of plantar fasciitis from these kinds of studies, you will be able to get enough information to tell someone about how long their plantar fasciitis might last after they start treatment for it. So, here are the results of the best studies done in this area that have really long follow-up periods:

Study #1

- the data of 100 patients were reviewed (Wolgin 1994)
- patients were followed for *at least* two years
- average follow-up was for forty-seven months
- 82 out of the 100 patients recovered *completely*, which took an average of 5.7 months from the start of treatment

Study #2

- the charts of 105 patients were reviewed (Davis 1994)
- patients were followed for *at least* two years
- average follow-up was for twenty-nine months
- 66 out of 105 patients recovered *completely*, which took an average of 5.1 months from the start of treatment.
- another 28 patients had only occasional mild discomfort
- thus, 94 out of 105 patients had a successful outcome

This is good news. While it does take months to recover *completely*, plantar fasciitis does not go on forever!

The point: Based on studies that have followed large groups of patients over extended periods of time, we can confidently say that most people with plantar fasciitis will, on average, recover completely around five months *after* starting treatment.

So now we have a general time frame. While we're looking at these studies, it would also be of interest to find out exactly what were the most effective treatments they used that enabled their patients to finally lick this painful condition. Let's take a look at study number two first:

Study #2

- relative rest/decrease current exercise
- anti-inflammatory medications
- heel cushion
- calf stretching exercises
- occasional steroid injections
- walking program if not regularly exercising
- custom foot insert if felt indicated

As you can see, the patients in this study received more than one treatment. But here's the problem you run into when trying to figure out the most effective treatment for plantar fasciitis from a study like this. If you give a patient five or six different treatments all at the same time, and their symptoms go away, there's really no way to tell for sure *which* treatment (or treatments) were the ones that did the trick. Therefore, we really can't tell much from this study in terms of what the best treatment(s) are for plantar fasciitis. All we can really say, is that if you have a patient do all that stuff above, the odds will be greatly stacked in their favor that they'll improve. Well, let's take a look at what the patients did in the first study to get better:

Study #1

- after being given options, patients generally chose their own treatments
- 66 tried stretching
- 64 tried cushioned inserts
- 51 tried anti-inflammatory medications
- 33 tried ice
- 31 tried injections
- 27 tried heat
- 9 tried a heel cup
- 3 tried a night splint
- 8 tried a walking program
- 3 tried plantar strapping
- 5 tried a hard orthotic
- 17 tried a shoe change

Interesting. 82 out of the 100 patients in this study recovered *completely*, despite the fact that subjects each chose different combinations of treatments *and* any given patient could have used more than one treatment at a time. If at this point, you're beginning to wonder if plantar fasciitis will get better over time no matter how you treat it, you're pretty much where I was at when I first went over these studies. So having this as my theory, I then proceeded to look up *all* the treatments for plantar fasciitis in the published literature that were tested out in *randomized controlled trials*. I'll go over these results in greater detail in a later chapter, as well as explain all about the randomized controlled trial, but for now, just know that these kinds of trials provide the highest form of proof in medicine that a treatment actually works. Now if my hunch was indeed correct–that the majority of plantar fasciitis patients will get better no matter what kind of treatment they get–then the studies should tell the tale. Here's a sample of what I found:

- one randomized controlled trial tested out shoe inserts to see if they could help plantar fasciitis sufferers (Landorf 2006). One group tried prefabricated shoe inserts, another group custom-fit inserts, and the last group a fake insert which provided little support to the foot. No other treatments were allowed during the study. At one year follow-up, *all three groups experienced improvements in pain and function with only small differences between the groups.*

- another randomized controlled trial tested out extracorporeal shock wave therapy (Speed 2003), a popular form of therapy commonly used in the treatment of tendonitis. In this study, one group of plantar fasciitis sufferers received active shock wave therapy, while another group received a fake treatment. Each group was treated once a month for 3 months. No other treatments were permitted during the study. At the end of the study, *both groups showed improvement with no significant differences existing between the two.*

- in this randomized controlled trial, the effectiveness of stretching was tested out for the short-term treatment of plantar fasciitis (Radford 2007). One group stretched their calf muscles daily and received a fake ultrasound treatment (sound waves designed to speed up healing), while another group just got the fake ultrasound. Once again, follow-up showed that *both groups improved over the two week period, with no differences between groups.*

I could go on and on, and quote many more studies, each testing out various treatments for plantar fasciitis, but the literature is very consistent in what it shows. The vast majority, and I mean *the vast majority* of randomized controlled trials, show that plantar fasciitis patients get better no matter which treatment group they get put into. For example, in the above studies, patients got better if they tried fancy custom shoe inserts or the fake inserts. They even got better if they got *fake* ultrasound treatments or *real* shock wave therapy!

The point: Plantar fasciitis is a condition that tends to improve regardless of which medical treatment is chosen. This also lends support to the idea that the natural history of plantar fasciitis is favorable.

So now that we know that the outlook is good for people with plantar fasciitis, and the prognosis favorable once treatment is started, we'll want to aim for the treament that is the cheapest, easiest, and most convenient to use.

Summary

✓ unlike other medical conditions, there are no natural history studies that have been done on plantar fasciitis. Therefore, its natural course is unknown.

✓ since we do have long term follow-up studies on plantar fasciitis patients that have gotten medical treatment, we can say that on average, plantar fasciitis improves around 5 months *after starting treatment*

✓ well-done studies that have tested the effectiveness of various treatments for plantar fasciitis show that it is a condition that seems to get better no matter what particular treatment option is used

✓ the fact that plantar fasciitis sufferers get better over time, no matter what particular treatment option is chosen, lends support to the idea that the natural history of plantar fasciitis is favorable

Chapter Three

The 5-Minute Plantar Fasciitis Solution

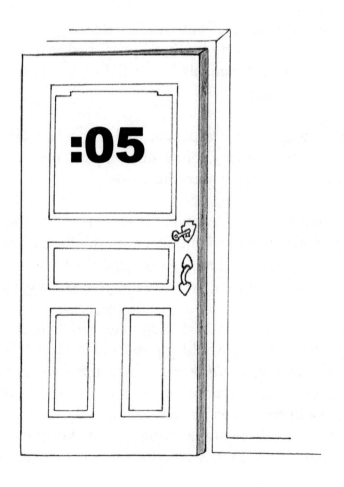

:05 | The 5-Minute Plantar Fasciitis Solution

"Proven pain relief," say the television commercials. "Shown to be effective" reads the medicine bottle. It sounds good, and is exactly what people want to hear, but how do you *really* know it's true?

In a word, research. If you want to know if a treatment for a problem, any condition really, is truly effective, the *only* way you can know for sure is to find out the results of any studies that have properly tested out the treatment. And, if the study has been published in a peer-reviewed journal, meaning that other professionals in the field have read it first and think it's fit to print, all the better.

So what exactly should a person look for when digging around in the research? I mean in today's information age, there are literally *piles* of studies readily accessible at your fingertips.

Well, in medicine, we have what is known as *the randomized controlled trial*. This research method produces the highest form of proof showing whether or not a treatment really works and it's what you'll want to look for first–since it's the best of the best. Let me give you a basic example.

Say you want to prove that magnetic shoe inserts get rid of plantar fasciitis. Well, first you would go out and find, maybe, 100 people with plantar fasciits and then *randomize* them into two groups of fifty–which means you pick them at random to go into one group or the other. Doing things this way keeps things fair because it makes sure that each subject has an equal chance at being put into either group–which makes sure that no one is purposely put here or there where they might do better or worse.

Next, you make one group the treatment group (meaning that they get to wear the magnetic shoe inserts) and the other one a control group (meaning that they get either a comparison treatment, or better yet, *no* treatment at all). Take note that the control group is one of the most important parts of the randomized controlled trial because it allows you to compare how people do when they *don't* get the treatment you're testing out.

Okay, so now you're ready to start your own randomized controlled trial and test out your theory that magnetic shoe inserts do indeed get rid of plantar fasciitis. You give the people in the treatment group their magnetic shoe inserts, let the people in the control group go about their normal business, and then check on everybody in, say, six weeks to see how their feet are doing. If, at the end of the six week trial, the magnetic shoe insert group has less pain than the control group, you can now say with confidence that magnetic shoe inserts are indeed an effective treatment for plantar fasciitis. That's because everyone at the start of the study had the same condition (plantar fasciitis), an equal chance of getting into either group, and the group that wore the magnetic shoe inserts were the only ones who got better. Therefore, we assume it must have been those inserts!

On the other hand, if the magnetic shoe insert group and control group both had the *same* amount of foot pain at the end of the six week study, then we would have to say that magnetic shoe inserts *don't* work at all, simply because all subjects ended up with the same amount of foot pain whether they wore a magnetic shoe insert or not. Pretty nifty set-up, huh?

At this point, some readers might be wondering just why I'm dragging them through all this research mumbo-jumbo. Well, it's not because I'm trying to turn you into junior scientists. No, it's for two *very* important reasons.

The first one is so that you will have every confidence that the 5-Minute Plantar Fasciits Solution really *does* work. Now that you know what a randomized controlled trial is, and that it produces the highest form of proof in medicine that a treatment is really effective, it will mean much more to you when I say that the treatment tools used in the 5-Minute Plantar Fasciitis Solution has been shown in randomized controlled trials to effectively decrease the symptoms of chronic plantar fasciitis. Unfortunately, I doubt you'll find too many other pain books on the self-help bookshelf that are based on this kind of evidence.

The second reason? Well, I guess the teacher in me likes to educate people about the randomized controlled trial so that they will become more informed consumers. If you're like me, you work at least forty hours a week and quite possibly have a family to take care of. We all work hard for our money and I think it's really unfair when someone asks us to spend some of it on a product or service that makes miraculous claims without a shred of real evidence!

However, now that *you* know exactly what to look for when deciding on a treatment for a particular problem (one or more randomized controlled trials that show effectiveness), you'll be able to tell if it's something you want to invest your time and money in, or if it's clearly a hit or miss venture.

A Tale of Two Stretches

In the last chapter, you learned that plantar fasciitis is a condition that can respond to a wide variety of treatments. Therefore, readers of this book, who most likely have suffered with plantar fasciitis for quite some time, will be looking for the ideal treatment that is cheap, convenient to do, and proven to work on *chronic* sufferers in randomized controlled trials. The 5-Minute Plantar Fasciitis Solution fulfills all of these requirements.

Now the treatment that makes up the 5-Minute Plantar Fasciitis Solution is based upon several well-done studies conducted at Ithaca College at the University of Rochester Campus. In the first study (DiGiovanni 2003), researchers chose to tackle the worst of the worst when it comes to plantar fasciitis patients–*long-term* sufferers who had been struggled with the condition for at least ten months. Truly a tough bunch to tackle, these 101 subjects were randomized into one of two groups:

- "Group A" which specifically stretched their plantar fascia 10 times, three times a day

    or

- "Group B" which specifically stretched their Achilles tendon (calf muscles) 10 times, three times a day

Additionally, *both* groups received over-the-counter, prefabricated full-length insoles, a three-week course of a non-steroidal anti-inflammatory medication, and viewed an educational video about plantar fasciitis. Patients were also instructed to discontinue all other treatments for heel pain and encouraged not to change their shoe wear or activity level.

So what happened at the end of the study some eight-weeks later? Well, in keeping with what we know about plantar fasciitis responding favorably to a wide variety of treatments, *both* groups reported an overall decrease in pain levels compared to the begining of the study–no big surprise there. However what was quite notable, was the fact that subjects in Group A (who specifically stretched their plantar fascia) were found to have *superior* results. Not only did these folks report having less pain than Group B, but they also had less activity limitations and were found to be significantly more satisfied after eight-weeks. Apparently all stretching is not created equal.

Now let's stop and think about this for a minute. We have two groups of plantar fasciitis sufferers who had been suffering for *at least* ten months, with a fair share of participants in the study actually struggling *for more than three years*.

Additionally, all participants in the study had failed many popular forms of therapy in the past, treatments such as anti-inflammatory medications, shoe inserts, heel cups, exercises, night splints, injections, and so on. Then, after only eight-weeks of stretching, both groups improve, one more than the other. What an impressive result! But hold on, that's not where the story ends...

Being clever researchers, this group then decided to take things one step further (DiGiovanni 2006). Recall that at the end of the first study, subjects who stretched their plantar fascia (Group A) fared much better than those that stretched their calf muscles (Group B). In other words, while improved, which was no small feat in and of itself, the people that did the traditional calf stretching simply *never* caught up symptom-wise to the people who specifically stretched their plantar fascia. Now, however, they were going to get their chance.

So, at the end of the first study, all participants who just did the calf stretching in Group B were now instructed to *stop* doing that stretch and *start* doing the specific plantar fascia stretch that produced the superior results in Group A. This was to continue for at least eight-weeks, and after that, subjects could just do the stretch as needed.

The researchers let *two years* pass. They then re-evaluated everyone they could (Group A *and* Group B) that had participated in original study to see how everyone fared over the long run. Let it be noted that this is another factor that makes this a truly rare plantar fasciitis study. While some randomized controlled trials show a clear benefit of one treatment over another one, you also want to know if at all possible, "How long did the treatment effects last?" For instance, did patients get better and stay better, or did they get better only to have the pain return in a month or two after the study ended? Of course one wouldn't have a clue unless subjects were followed for an extended period of time. That's why the *best* randomized controlled trials, such as this one, have a sizeable follow-up period, such as a year or two. Anyway, how do you suppose all the subjects in the study, who had suffered with plantar fasciitis for months, some for years, were doing *two years* after starting a simple plantar fascia stretching routine?

If you said that both groups were doing *the same* at the two-year follow-up evaluation, you're right on the money! In other words, even those subjects in Group B that started out doing the calf stretch, and then switched to the plantar fasciitis stretch, ended up doing just as well as those in Group A who stretched their plantar fascia from the start. Here's a few details of how things turned out for *both* groups at the two-year follow-up when all was said and done:

- 92% reported total satisfaction or satisfaction with minor reservations

- 94% reported a decrease in pain with 58% having *no* pain

- 77% reported no limitation in recreational activities or activities of daily living

- 62% of subjects achieved the best results within six months after starting the plantar fascia stretch

- no patients ended up needing surgery

Some readers may be wondering at this point, "Could the anti-inflammatory medications or shoe insoles given at the beginning of the study have anything to do with the patient's pain relief?" Of course they could, and it would have been an almost perfect study if the two stretches *alone* would have just been tested. However, if the shoe inserts and medications *did* significantly help relieve symptoms, both groups would have been affected equally because both groups got them—which takes their effects "out of the picture" so to speak.

Keep in mind that both groups were given the *exact* same treatment protocol in the beginning, except that one group did the calf stretch and the other the plantar fascia stretch. And since one group did better than the other, that being the plantar fascia stretching group, the only variable that could account for this difference would most likely be the type of stretch performed.

The 5-Minute Plantar Fasciitis Solution

As you might have already guessed, the 5-minute Plantar Fasciitis Solution involves stretching. However, it's probably unlike any kind of stretching you've ever done before *because this stretch precisely targets the plantar fascia.* Developed by the authors of the studies we've just been discussing, it goes like this:

Step One

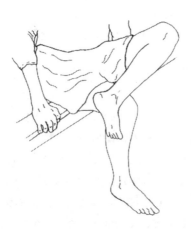

1. Find a comfortable place to sit.
2. Get into the above position. The foot you want to stretch should be on top. In the above picture, the *left* foot is about to be stretched.

Step Two

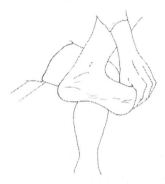

1. Place your fingers across *the base* of your toes like the above picture
2. Next, pull the toes back towards the shin until a stretch is felt in the arch or plantar fascia. Hold 10 seconds.

Step Three

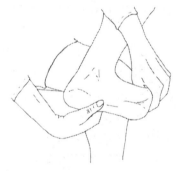

1. When doing it correctly, you should feel tension in your plantar fascia when you press on it. In the above picture, the right thumb is pressing in and checking for tension.

Just as important as actually doing the stretch itself, is *strictly* following these guidelines to a 'T':

- hold the stretch for a *full* 10 seconds
- repeat the stretch 10 times in a row
- do this three times a day
- the first set of stretching **must** be done *before* taking your first step in the morning
- if you have been sitting for a prolonged period of time, perform the stretch *before* you stand up

And that's it! A quick calculation reveals that readers should spend a total of about five minutes a day stretching. This is because ten 10-second stretches performed for a total of 30 times a day works out to 300 seconds– *or* five minutes.

Keep in mind that while this simple stretch may seem almost *too* easy to be of any help, it has been *proven* to work in randomized controlled trials on long-term plantar fasciitis sufferers when nothing else would do the trick. *But, you've got to stretch correctly and follow the above guidelines.*

Especially key to making the stretching work is to make absolutely sure that you do it *before standing up* after you've been off your feet for a while, for example when you first get out of bed in the morning or when you have been sitting for a long time. As most plantar fasciitis sufferers can tell you, those first few steps you take after you've been off your feet for awhile are quite painful. Stretching out the plantar fascia *before* putting weight on it makes things much easier on the fascia, eliminates further trauma to it, and creates an environment where it can finally begin to heal. To remind you of this and improve your consistency, I've included some stretching logs in Chapter 7 to help readers keep track of their stretching each day.

How Fast Does It Work?

I always hesitate to throw out numbers as people inevitably start to worry if their recovery doesn't follow the "normal" pattern. *However*, if forced to pin down a time frame, I'd have to say that on average, most people can expect significant improvement within the first four to eight weeks of starting the program.

How Long Do I Continue Stretching?

Everyone needs to continue with the plantar fascia stretch for at least eight full weeks–period. At that point:

- *if your plantar fasciitis is gone*, do the stretch periodically (i.e. several times a week) for maintenance. Note that this number is based on clinical experience as there are no studies yet to tell us the optimal number of times one needs to stretch in order to prevent a relapse.

- *if your symptoms are better, but not quite gone yet*, then continue with the stretching. Best results are usually reached within a six month period.

- *if you've noted no change in symptoms*, then stretching is not the answer. Consult your doctor and consider trying one of the alternative treatments in Chapter Six.

You now have all the tools and information you need to get started. And as you proceed, just remember, plantar fasciitis is *not* a condition that was created overnight–and it won't go away overnight either. Be patient. Each day of stretching brings you one step closer to eliminating your symptoms.

Summary

✓ the randomized controlled trial is the highest form of proof in medicine that a treatment is effective and works

✓ specifically stretching the plantar fascia has been shown in randomized controlled trials to help long-term plantar fasciitis sufferers that have failed other treatments

✓ the 5-Minute Plantar Fasciitis Solution involves targeted stretching of the plantar fascia for a total of five minutes a day

✓ one of the most important things to remember is to stretch the plantar fascia *before* you put weight on your foot if you've been off it for awhile

✓ the majority of patients get significant relief in four to eight weeks after starting the stretching, with best results usually achieved within a six month period

Chapter Four

Measuring Your Progress

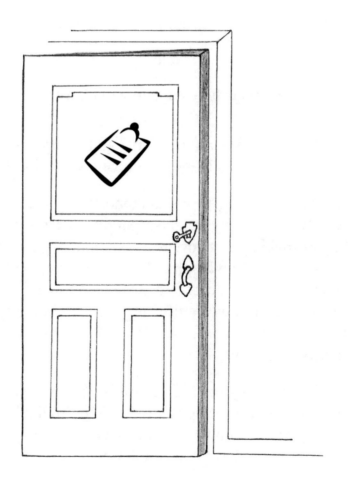

Measuring Your Progress

Okay. You've learned all about the plantar fascia, have started the stretching, and are on the road to recovery. So now what should you expect?

Well, we all know you should expect to get better. But what exactly does *better* mean? As a physical therapist treating patients, it means two distinct things to me:

- your foot starts to *feel* better

    and

- your foot starts to *work* better

And so, when a patient returns for a follow-up visit, I re-assess them, looking for specific changes in their foot pain, as well as their foot function.

In this book, I'm going to recommend that readers do the same thing periodically. Why? Simply because people in pain can't always see the progress they're making. For instance sometimes a person's pain is exactly the same, but they aren't aware that they can now actually do some motions or tasks that they couldn't do before–a sure sign that things are healing. *Or*, sometimes a person still has significant foot pain but they're not aware that it's actually occurring less frequently–yet another good indication that positive changes are taking place.

Whatever the case may be, if a person isn't looking at the bigger picture, and doesn't think they're getting any better, they're likely to get discouraged and stop doing the 5-Minute Plantar Fasciitis Solution altogether–even though they really might have been on the right track.

On the other hand though, what if you periodically check your progress and are keenly aware that your foot has made some changes for the better? What if you can *positively* see objective results? My guess is that you're going to be giving yourself a healthy dose of motivation to keep on truckin' with the stretching.

Having said that, I'm going to show you exactly what to check for from time to time so that you can monitor *all* the changes that are taking place in your foot. I call them "outcomes" and there are two of them.

Outcome #1:
Look for Changes in Your Pain

First of all, you should look for changes in your pain. I know this may sound silly, but sometimes it's my job to get a person to see that their pain *is* actually improving. You see, a lot of people come to physical therapy thinking they're going to be pain-free right away. Then, when they're not instantly better and still having pain, they often start to worry and become discouraged. Truth is, I have seen very few people start doing a stretch and get instantly better. Better yes, but not *instantly* better.

Over the years, I have found that patients usually respond to therapy in a quite predictable pattern. One of three things will almost always occur as a person begins to turn the corner and get better:

- your foot pain is just as intense as always, however now it is occurring much less frequently

or

- your foot pain is now *less* intense, even though it still occurring just as frequently

or

- you start to notice less intense foot pain *and* it is now occurring less frequently

The point here is to make sure that you keep a sharp eye out for these three scenarios as you continue using the 5-Minute Plantar Fasciitis Solution. If *any* of them occur, it will be a sure sign that the specific plantar fascia stretching is helping. You can then look forward to the pain gradually getting better, usually over the weeks to come.

Outcome #2:
Look for Changes in Foot Function

Looking at how well your foot works is very important because sometimes foot function improves *before* the pain does. For example, sometimes a patient will do the stretching for a while, and although their foot will still hurt a lot, they are able to do many activities that they haven't been able to in a while–a really good indicator that healing is taking place *and* that the pain should be easing up soon.

While measuring your foot function may sound like a pain in the butt, it doesn't have to be. In this book, I'm recommending that readers use a quick and easy assessment tool known as *The Lower Extremity Functional Scale.*

The Lower Extremity Functional Scale has actually been around for awhile and has been used to document disability in plantar fasciitis patients (Riddle 2004). It is well researched (Binkley 1999, Martin 2007) and has been shown to be:

- *valid* (it actually measures what it's suppose to be measuring)

- *reliable* (you can get the same result with repeated testing)

- *responsive* (has the ability to detect changes in a person over time)

Additionally, the Lower Extremity Functional Scale takes about 3 minutes to complete and can be scored without a calculator in under a minute. Now that's my kinda test!

So what exactly does taking the Lower Extremity Functional Scale involve? Not much. You simply go down a list of twenty commonly performed activities, circling the number to the right which indicates how difficult it is for you to do them *because of your plantar fasciitis*. Then, when you've done that, you simply add up the numbers you circled and see how many you have out of a possible 80 points.

What does the number mean? Well, 80 is the highest number you can score on the Lower Extremity Functional Scale, and when you achieve this, it means that you are functioning at a high level *without* much interference from your plantar fasciitis. On the other hand, a lower score indicates that plantar fasciitis *is* keeping you from doing many everyday tasks. On the next page is the scale.

The Lower Extremity Functional Scale

We are interested in knowing whether you are having any difficulty at all with the activities listed below because of your lower limb problem for which you are currently seeking attention. Please provide an answer for **each** activity.

Today, do you or would you have any difficulty at all with:

(Circle one number on each line)

Activities	Extreme Difficulty or Unable to Perform Activity	Quite a Bit of Difficulty	A Little Moderate Difficulty	Bit of Difficulty	No Difficulty
a. Any of your usual work, housework or school activities	0	1	2	3	4
b. Your usual hobbies, recreational or sporting activities	0	1	2	3	4
c. Getting into or out of the bath	0	1	2	3	4
d. Walking between rooms	0	1	2	3	4
e. Putting on your shoes or socks	0	1	2	3	4
f. Squatting	0	1	2	3	4
g. Lifting an object, like a bag of groceries from the floor	0	1	2	3	4
h. Performing light activities around your home	0	1	2	3	4
i. Performing heavy activities around your home	0	1	2	3	4
j. Getting into or out of a car	0	1	2	3	4
k. Walking 2 blocks	0	1	2	3	4
l. Walking a mile	0	1	2	3	4
m. Going up or down 10 stairs (about 1 flight of stairs)	0	1	2	3	4
n. Standing for 1 hour.	0	1	2	3	4
o. Sitting for 1 hour	0	1	2	3	4
p. Running on even ground	0	1	2	3	4
q. Running on uneven ground	0	1	2	3	4
r. Making sharp turns while running fast	0	1	2	3	4
s. Hopping	0	1	2	3	4
t. Rolling over in bed	0	1	2	3	4

Now, add up all of the numbers you circled and write the total here ⟶ ___/80
The more out of 80 you have, the better, with 80/80 being a perfect score.

*The Lower Extremity Functional Scale above is adapted from Physical Therapy 1999;79:371-383.

So how did you do? Remember, the higher the number, the better your function–which is what you want to shoot for. If you scored 80, you probably don't need this book too much. On the other hand, lower scores, such as 9/80 or 15/80, show us that your plantar fasciitis is *really* limiting your activities. If you did score this low, don't worry. Just keep taking the Lower Extremity Functional Scale every few weeks or so, and as you continue with the stretching, you should see your score go up and up as time passes. Remember, often times foot function gets better *before* the pain does.

Summary

✓ being aware of your progress is a key part of treating your own plantar fasciitis–it motivates you to keep doing the stretching

✓ look for the pain to become less *intense*, less *frequent*, or both to let you know that the 5-Minute Plantar Fasciitis Solution is working

✓ sometimes a foot starts to work better *before* it starts to feel better. Taking the Lower Extremity Functional Scale from time-to-time makes you aware of improving foot function.

Chapter Five

How to Keep Plantar Fasciitis From Coming Back

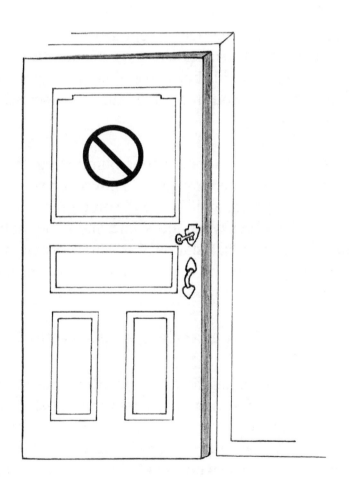

How to Keep Plantar Fasciitis From Coming Back

Okay, let's take out our crystal ball for a moment. Pretend that after reading this book, you follow the 5-Minute Plantar Fasciitis Solution exactly as instructed, and over time, your symptoms go *completely* away.

Is that it? End of story? Well, it could be. But while it is true that plantar fasciitis does *not* have a particular reputation for coming back around to getcha again, there is of course, always a chance that it *could* come back. And that's why I feel like this book would be incomplete unless I took some time out to briefly talk about the things that can increase one's chances of getting plantar fasciitis.

Now we're not really talking about eliminating the *causes* of plantar fasciitis, simply because nobody really knows for sure what causes it. We have some logical guesses, and I've read some great biomechanical theories in the literature. However when all is said and done, nobody can really say with absolute certainty what started the whole problem in the first place. Therefore, we're going to be concentrating more on eliminating the *risk factors* for getting plantar fasciitis.

What exactly is a risk factor?

A risk factor is something that can increase a person's chance of getting a disease or condition. For example, smoking is a risk factor for getting lung cancer–if you smoke, you have a higher chance of getting cancer. This does *not* mean, however, that everybody who smokes will absolutely get lung cancer, since there are those who smoke that don't ever get the disease.

Keep this in mind when we talk about risk factors and plantar fasciitis. These are just characteristics that have been shown in the research that will *increase* your odds of getting plantar fasciitis, but having them does not guarantee in any way that you will absolutely get it.

By the same token, *eliminating as many risk factors as you can will decrease your chances of getting plantar fasciitis*–which is the whole point of this chapter.

How do we determine the risk factors for getting plantar fasciitis?

While my goal here is not to turn you into junior researchers, I feel like it's important to spend a page or two talking about how risk factors are determined. This is because there are a lot of myths and misconceptions out there as to what the risk factors for plantar fasciitis *really* are. Since many readers no doubt have heard or read many different things, I'm going to give you the correct, research-based information–and I want you to know how I got it.

Now one of the most powerful ways to determine a risk factor is to conduct an experiment. Using plantar fasciitis for our example, one would generally go like this:

- a bunch of people *without* plantar fasciitis are randomly divided into two groups
- one group gets exposed to the risk factor in question, let's say high-heeled shoes, and the other is not; otherwise, both groups are treated exactly the same
- the two groups are observed over time
- if the group that wore the high heeled shoes ends up having a higher rate of plantar fasciitis than the other group, we could say that wearing high heeled shoes could be considered a risk factor for getting plantar fasciitis

While this is one of the best ways of determining a risk factor, there aren't many of these kinds of studies around for good reasons. A big one is that it's just not ethical in many cases to impose possible risk factors on healthy people for the sake of science. I mean, would you want to be in the group that had to wear the high heels and take a chance on getting plantar fasciitis? Not too surprisingly, no such experimental studies have been done on plantar fasciitis.

So, the next best thing we've got is *the observational study*. Most studies of risk are observational and are called this simply because the researcher is watching or *observing* groups of people in an attempt to find a link between some characteristic and a disease. While there are many different kinds, we're going to discuss three types: *prospective*, *retrospective*, and *case-control* studies. Here's a basic example of each in which I'm pretending to find out if being overweight is a risk factor for getting plantar fasciitis:

- *prospective*–this is where I would go out and recruit a group of people **without** plantar fasciitis and weigh them. Then I would follow them over time to see who ends up getting plantar fasciitis in the long run and who doesn't. If more of the overweight people ended up getting plantar fasciitis compared to the rest of the group, then this would lend support to the idea that being overweight is a risk factor for getting plantar fasciitis.

- *retrospective*–say I had trouble putting together a group of people **without** plantar fasciitis to follow. Well, I could always look *back* (retrospectively) at a bunch of medical records and do the same thing as the above. This would mean digging up a set of *old* medical records of people who didn't have plantar fasciitis at some point in time, checking to see how much each person weighed, and then finding out who did or didn't end up getting plantar fasciitis over time. I could then look for any link between being overweight and getting plantar fasciitis.

- *case-control*–in this type of study, I would find a group of people **with** plantar fasciitis and another group of people **without** it. This could be done by either recruiting people or looking at medical records. I would then compare the two groups to see if people with plantar fasciitis really do weigh more than people without it.

Keep in mind that these are just **basic** descriptions of how some observational studies work. My main goal here is to just give you a general idea of how they are conducted without getting you too bogged down in details. And with this knowledge, you'll not only better understand how some of the studies in this chapter were carried out, but you'll also know what makes up a good risk factor study for *any* medical condition you might hear or read about in the future.

Now after looking at the various types of observational studies, hopefully you noticed one thing–they all compare *two* groups in order to determine a risk factor. While this may seem to be just common sense, I have come across many instances where something like having a high arch was said to be a risk factor for plantar fasciitis based on observing only *one* group of people. Let me give you an example:

- a researcher conducts a study where he has taken 50 patients with plantar fasciitis, measured their foot arches, and noticed that 30 of them have high arches. He concludes that having a high arch is a risk factor for getting plantar fasciitis and publishes the results. People who read the research article start to think the same thing.

While this seems like logical thinking, it's really a *very* poor way to come to the conclusion that something is a risk factor. The main flaw here is that the researcher is only looking at *one* group of people–patients that have plantar fasciitis. And while it's true that he has found a large number of high arches in patients with plantar fasciitis, the numbers mean little because he doesn't know how common high arches are in people *without* plantar fasciitis. It is only when one compares the number of high arches in people **with** plantar fasciitis, to the number of high arches in people **without** plantar fasciitis, that you would be able to see if there was a difference between the two and conclude that high arches are indeed a real risk factor. Once again, this may be seem like common sense to many readers, but you will find a lot of this kind of logic floating around in various articles as well as the clinic.

While it's great to try and make associations between two things based upon everyday observations, which is exactly how ideas behind great studies get started, just remember that they are only *theories* until properly tested out in well-done research studies.

The point: Eliminating risk factors will go a long way in decreasing your chances of getting plantar fasciitis. Make sure you aren't wasting your time and effort worrying about risk factors that are based on hearsay or poor research.

The Risk Factors

Okay, now that you have a little background as to how risk factors are correctly determined, it's time to get down to discussing them. Please note that in this section, we will be talking only about studies that were done on *non-athletes*, and therefore, the risk factors listed will pertain the best to people who engage in your average, everyday activities.

The Big Three

One of the best studies ever conducted on the risk factors for plantar fasciitis comes from the Virginia Commonwealth University in Richmond Virginia. It was there that researchers put together a group of patients that had plantar fasciitis, and then compared them to a control group with no foot problems. Additionally, and what makes this a *really* good study, is the fact that the people in the control group were matched to the plantar fasciitis patients by age and sex. This means, for example, that if researchers had a 40 year-old man with plantar fasciitis, they went out and found another 40-year old man *without* plantar fasciitis to compare him to. Now that's what I call good research! While the study looked at many factors that could be linked to getting plantar fasciitis, only three stood out:

- weighing too much
- spending a lot of time on your feet
- not having a flexible ankle

At this point, many readers are probably wondering, "How much weight is too much weight?" or "Exactly how flexible should my ankle be?" Soooo, let's go over each one quickly…

Weighing Too Much

Weighing too much can mean many things to many people. While there is definitely more than one way to classify a person as weighing too much, many research studies, as well as the one above, use what is called the *body mass index.* The body mass index, or more commonly known as "the BMI", is simply a number that is calculated from a person's height and weight. It is a reliable indicator of body fatness for people, and although the BMI does not measure body fat directly, research has shown that it does correlate to more sophisticated measures of body fat, such as underwater weighing.

Additionally, the BMI is inexpensive and easy-to-perform. To find out your BMI, grab any simple calculator and follow these three easy steps:

1. Multiply your weight in pounds by 705.

2. Divide your answer by your height in inches.

3. Now divide this answer by your height in inches again.

The result is your BMI.

Pretty easy, huh? Now here's a real-life example to make sure you're on the right track. Let's say that you're 5'6'' (66 inches) and you weigh 185 pounds:

185 multiplied by 705 = 130,425

130,425 divided by 66 = 1,976.14

1,976.14 divided by 66 = 29.94, or a BMI of 29.9

Okay, enough math. Now that you've got your own personal BMI number, what does it mean? Well…

If your BMI is below 18.5…. you're underweight

If your BMI is 18.5 to 24.9… you're in the ideal range

If your BMI is 25 to 29.9…... you're overweight

If your BMI is 30 or higher… you're obese

In the study done at the Virginia Commonwealth University, researchers found that as far as weight is concerned, having a BMI of *more than 30* put people at the highest for the development of plantar fasciitis. Other controlled studies also support the link between increased body weight and plantar fasciitis (Prichasuk 1994).

Since it is beyond the scope of this book to get into detailed weight loss strategies, readers who need a little work in this area are referred to one of my other books, *"The No-Beach, No-Zone, No-Nonsense Weight Loss Plan, A Pocket Guide to What Works."* My hope in writing it was to put a handy, evidence-based book on weight loss into the hands of readers who specifically need to lose weight for orthopaedic and other health reasons. It is the result of a literature review I did of the last 45-plus years of weight loss research and contains only practical strategies that have been proven to work in randomized controlled trials. Consulting a medical professional with expertise in weight loss, such as a nutritionist, is also highly recommended.

Spending a Lot of Time on Your Feet

In the Virginia Commonwealth University study, no data was collected as to the actual number of hours that study participants spent on their feet during the day. Instead, researchers simply asked the question, "Do you spend the majority of your workday on your feet?" It was found that if one answered "yes" to this question, then they had a significantly increased risk of plantar fasciitis.

Unfortunately, in terms of realistically getting off your feet more during the day, there are only a few options available to most people–either change jobs, or modify the one you have. Therefore, becoming more aware of how long you're actually on your feet and trying to sit when possible, even for brief periods to break things up, is probably the most practical strategy to try.

Not Having a Flexible Ankle

Of the three risk factors that were identified in the study, having tightness in the ankle joint was found to be the most important. Specifically, researchers found that the tighter a person's ankle was when they pulled their foot *up*, the more at risk they were to get plantar fasciitis. In medicine, this foot motion is referred to as *dorsiflexion*. Here's a picture of what it looks like:

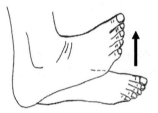

Figure 3.1 Pulling your foot up is a motion known as dorsiflexion

How tight is tight enough to put you at risk? Well, to answer this, I need to first show you how we measure dorsiflexion–then you can check your own feet to see if they have good motion or not. So, here's a picture of what your foot looks like when it's in the position of *zero degrees of dorsiflexion*:

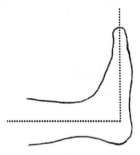

Figure 3.2 This foot is in zero degrees of dorsiflexion.

As you can see, when your foot is at zero degrees of dorsiflexion, it looks kind of like an "L" shape or a right angle. Now using this position as a frame of reference, let's take a look at your own feet to see how tight you are:

1. First, sit on the floor with your knees out *straight*. Using your arms to prop yourself up is okay.

2. Now have a friend gently push one of your feet up towards your head (which is the motion of dorsiflexion). This is done by applying pressure just under the toes on the ball of your foot.

3. Have your friend continue to push your foot up as high up as it will comfortably go. You will feel a stretch on the back of your leg in the area of your calf muscle.

4. When your foot can comfortably go up no further, hold this position for a second and look at the angle of your foot from the side. What do you and your friend see?

    -   if you *couldn't even* get your foot up to the zero degrees of dorsiflexion position, as in picture 3.2, your ankle motion puts you at risk to get plantar fasciitis

    -   if you could *only* get your foot up to the zero degrees of dorsiflexion position, as in picture 3.2, and no higher, your ankle motion puts you at risk to get plantar fasciitis

    -   if you can get your foot up to the the zero degrees of dorsiflexion position *plus eleven degrees higher or more,* your ankle motion *does not* put you at risk to get plantar fasciitis. A foot in the position of 11 degrees of dorsiflexion looks something like this:

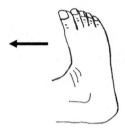

Figure 3.3 With the leg on the floor, this foot is
approximately pulled up into the position of eleven
degrees of dorsiflexion. *Any* ankle position lower
than this one puts you at risk to get plantar fasciitis.

> ***The bottom line:*** If your friend can push your foot up to the
> the zero degrees of dorsiflexion position *plus eleven degrees*
> *higher or more*, your ankle flexibility does not put you at risk to
> get plantar fasciitis. If your friend *can't* push your foot up to
> this position, then your are at risk.

Now keep in mind that when it comes to figuring out how flexible your
ankle is, this is about as good as you're going to be able to do on your own.
Granted it's not the most precise way, but it's purpose is to give you a
general idea if you have significant tightness in your ankle that is putting
you at risk for getting plantar fasciitis. Know too that the best way of getting
an accurate assessment of your ankle range of motion is to have it
professionally measured by a physical therapist (or other health professional)
using what is called a *goniometer*.

So how'd you do? If you didn't quite make it to the eleven degrees of
dorsiflexion position, then the remedy is to stretch out your ankles in order
to make them more flexible and decrease your risk of getting plantar
fasciitis. While there are many different techniques to choose from when it
comes to getting stretched out, by far the easiest and least complicated way
is what is known as *the static stretch.* A static (or stationary) stretch takes a
tight muscle, puts it in a lengthened position, and keeps it there for a certain
period of time. For instance, if you wanted to use the static stretch technique

to make the hamstring muscle on the back of your thigh more flexible, you could simply bend over with your knees straight and try to touch your toes. Thus, as you are holding this position, the muscle is being *statically stretched*. There's no bouncing, just a gentle, sustained stretch. But how much stretching does one really need to do in order to get rid of a tight ankle?

To answer that question, we need do what we've always done to get to the correct information–see what the research has to say about things. By finding out what has already been proven to be effective, we avoid wasting our valuable time and effort merely "trying out" methods that may or may not really work. So, here are the results of a literature search I did one time when I was looking for all the randomized controlled trials that compared people who statically stretched their calf muscles to increase dorsiflexion, to a control group that did *no* stretching at all:

Randomized Controlled Trials Comparing Static Calf Muscle Stretching to No Stretching

study	stretch used	length of time stretch held for	# of times repeated	results
Gajdosik 2007	standing stretch	15 seconds	10 times/day, 5 days/week	gained 7° in 6 wks.
Gajdosik 2005	standing stretch	15 seconds	10 times/day, 3 days/week	gained 5.1° in 8 wks.
Pratt 2003	standing stretch	3 minutes	1 time/day, 3 days in a row	no gains noted
Youdas 2003	standing stretch	30 seconds 60 seconds 2 minutes	1 time/day, ≥ 5 days/week 1 time/day, ≥ 5 days/week 1 time/day, ≥ 5 days/week	no gains noted no gains noted no gains noted
Peres 2002	on stomach using a weighted pulley	10 minutes	1 time/day, 14 times in 3 wks	no change in net ROM
Knight 2001	standing stretch	20 seconds	4 times/day, 3 days/week	gained 6° in 6 wks.
Bohannon 1994	standing stretch	5 minutes	a one-time stretch	gained 2.3°

Glancing at our handy table, you can see that ankle flexibility can be significantly increased in a matter of weeks using a simple standing stretch. And, while you can use any of the stretching guidelines from the above studies that showed positive gains in ankle motion, it looks like the most efficient way to get the job done is to hold the stretch position for twenty seconds, do it four times daily, three days out of the week. Here are two standing stretches, just choose the one you like best:

The Stair Stretch

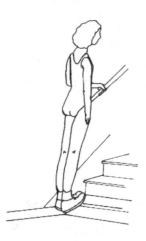

1. Find a step to stretch on, preferably one that has a rail next to it to hold on to.

2. Get into the stretch position as shown in the picture. You should have the front part of each foot (the ball of your foot) on the edge of the step. Both knees should be straight.

3. Now try to relax your leg muscles and let your heels sink down. At this point you should feel a good stretch in the back of your lower legs, not pain.

3. Hold this position for 20 seconds. Then rest for a few seconds. Repeat three more times.

4. Do the above three times a week with a day of rest in between (i.e. M-W-F *or* Tu-Th-Sa).

The Wall Stretch

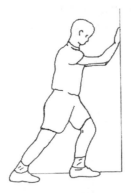

1. Find a wall that you can safely lean against.

2. Stand about 3 to 4 feet from the wall. Place your hands flat against the wall at shoulder level with your elbows straight.

3. Now step forward, bending the left knee, and shift your body weight forward onto the left leg. The right heel should remain **flat** on the floor with the knee straight. You should be in the same position as the above picture, which stretches the *right* ankle.

4. To stretch, simply continue to shift your weight forward slowly and gently, making sure you keep your right knee straight. Stop when your right heel just begins to rise off the floor. At this point, you should feel a good stretch in your right lower leg, not pain.

5. If you find that you're bumping into the wall as you shift your weight forward, just move both legs back a bit and then try shifting forward again.

3. Hold this position for 20 seconds. Then rest for a few seconds. Repeat three more times. Now switch legs and do the opposite to stretch the *left* ankle.

4. Do the above three times a week with a day of rest in between (i.e. stretch on M-W-F *or* Tu-Th-Sa)

What About Heel Spurs?

A heel spur is a "hook" of bone, that when found on an X-ray, occurs on the underside of a person's heel. Here's a picture to give you an idea of their general location on the foot:

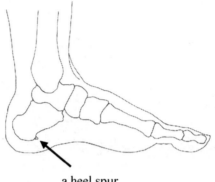

a heel spur.

The connection between heel spurs and plantar fasciitis is not entirely understood *or* as simple as some people would like to make it. For example, we now know that spurs forming within the attachment of the plantar fascia itself are actually very *uncommon* (Osborne 2006). Rather, the most frequent site of heel bone spurs occur at the attachments of small foot muscles, such as the flexor digitorum brevis (Forman 1990, McCarthy 1979).

To further complicate maters, there are many people with plantar fasciitis *that have* heel spurs, and many people with plantar fasciitis *that don't*. And then there's the fact that many people walk around everyday with heel spurs and no have pain. Take a look at the results of these studies and you'll see what I mean:

- an *X-ray* study found that 85% of subjects with plantar fasciitis had heel spurs compared to a rate of 46% in painfree subjects (Osborne 2006)

- an *ultrasound* study found that 31% of subjects with plantar fasciitis had heel spurs compared to a rate of 26% in painfree subjects (Akfirat 2003)

- an *MRI* study found that 50% of subjects with plantar fasciitis had heel spurs compared to a rate of 27% in painfree subjects (Berkowitz 1991)

As you can see from the above, although researchers *have* consistently found a higher rate of heel spurs in people with plantar fasciitis, there's hardly a clear-cut link between the two. Just take a look at the last study where half of the plantar fasciitis sufferers had heels spurs–which of course means that the other half *didn't* have them (Berkowitz 1991). Additionally, there are no randomized controlled trials showing that removing a heel spur will cure one from plantar fasciitis either. So, until more research is conducted and we know more, my advice is *not* to spend too much time worrying about them.

Are There Any Other Risk Factors I Should Know About?

None that have been supported enough in the published scientific literature for you to be worried about. For instance, one controlled observational study found that patients with plantar fasciitis had a thicker heel pad (the lump of fat on your heel that cushions your step) than normal subjects (Prichasuk 1994). While a noteworthy observation, I'm not really sure what to do with that little tidbit when it comes to decreasing one's chances of getting plantar fasciitis.

Then there's the research that looked at a possible link between the shape of your arch and plantar fasciitis:

- one study found that patients with plantar fasciitis had a flatter arch when compared to normal subjects (Prichasuk 1994). *However...*

- another study compared the arches of plantar fasciitis sufferers to the arches of control subjects which were matched for age, gender, and body weight (Wearing 2004). *No link was found between the shape of the foot arch and plantar fasciitis.*

And then there are a few studies that have looked at the flexibility of your big toe and its relationship to plantar fasciits:

- one study compared the big toe flexibility of a group of runners with plantar fasciitis to a group of runners *without* plantar fasciitis (Creighton 1987). Researchers found that runners suffering with plantar fasciitis had less flexibility in their big toes. *However...*

- another study measured the flexibility of the big toe in plantar fasciitis patients as well as in a control group that was matched for age and sex (Allen 2003). *Big toe flexibility did not differ between the two groups.*

As you can gather, if one looks at just the good stuff, that being observational studies that have included a comparison control group–which are basically the best kind of studies when it comes to determining risk factors–there are really only three major risk factors to be concerned about. However also keep in mind that research *is* always an ongoing process, and as more quality studies are done, we may indeed see more being added to this list.

Summary

✓ a risk factor is something that may increase a person's chance of getting a disease or condition

✓ having a risk factor, however, in no way guarantees that you will absolutely get a particular disease or condition

✓ eliminating as many plantar fasciitis risk factors as you can will decrease your chances of getting it

✓ observational studies *that have a control group* are some of the best ways to determine risk factors for getting plantar fasciitis

✓ there are three main risk factors for getting plantar fasciitis that stand out in the literature: weighing too much, spending a lot of time on your feet, and not having a flexible ankle

✓ the connection between heel spurs and plantar fasciitis is not entirely understood yet

✓ many people with plantar fasciitis have heel spurs, but then again, many people with plantar fasciitis do not. Furthermore, a lot of people walk around with heel spurs and *no pain*.

Chapter Six

Other Options For
Eliminating Plantar Fasciitis

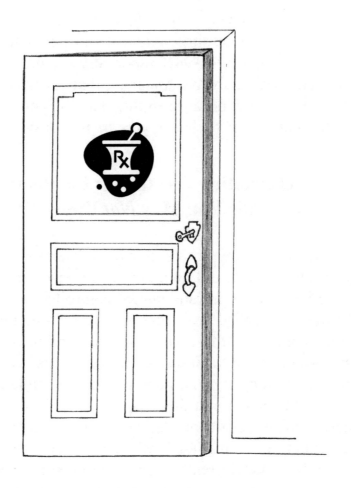

Other Options for Eliminating Plantar Fasciitis

After treating both in and outpatients with a wide variety of musculoskeletal conditions for over 16 years, I have come to realize that there is no single treatment for any given medical condition that will work for *every* patient, *all* the time, *without* fail. The 5-Minute Plantar Fasciitis Solution is no different.

While it *has* been shown to be effective in treating some of the most resistant cases of plantar fasciitis, and will no doubt help the majority of readers (recall that in the study 94% reported a decrease in pain), the fact of the matter is that there is always *someone*, that for whatever reason, *won't* get relief. But that's okay, because in this book, if you end up being one of those few, I'm not going to leave you in the dust. For you, we have options...

Alternative Treatments for Plantar Fasciitis You May *Not* Know About

What I've done for you in this chapter is summarize the results of an extensive literature search I did on all the treatments for plantar fasciitis that have shown to be effective in randomized controlled trials. It only includes those randomized controlled trials that have tested out a single treatment by itself, and then compared it to a control group and/or other treatments. For example, say we're trying to find out if shoe inserts relieve pain in plantar fasciitis patients. A study in which one group wore shoe inserts and another group didn't would make it into this chapter. On the other hand, a study that had volunteers wear shoe inserts *as well as* take anti-inflammatory medications would not be included. Why? Because one of the best ways to know if a specific treatment really works, is to test that treatment in a study by itself, *without* combining it with other treatments. By doing things this way, we can see how effective it and it alone really is.

As we've said in Chapter Three, the randomized controlled trial is the best of the best when it comes to proving that a treatment actually works, so what you've got here is a concise list of some of the most effective treatments around for plantar fasciitis. While many are nowhere as cheap or convenient to do as The 5-Minute Plantar Fasciitis Solution, they are great alternatives you and your doctor might want to talk about trying if all else fails.

shoe orthotics and insoles

Websters defines an orthotic as "a device (as a brace or splint) for supporting, immobilizing, or treating muscles, joints, or skeletal parts which are weak, ineffective, deformed, or injured." When it comes to the foot, an orthotic is usually thought of as some type of shoe insert that is intended to alter the way the foot sits in a shoe or moves while walking.

Since it has often been thought that plantar fasciitis is a condition that is caused by things such as high or low arches, it is no surprise that studies have tested out various shoe inserts to try and correct foot abnormalities to alleviate pain. Here's what some of the randomized controlled trials have to say about their effectiveness:

- one study had patients wear either a shoe insert made of soft thin foam, a pre-made firm foam insert, or a customized plastic insert (Landorf 2006). *All three groups experienced improvements in pain and function at 3 and 12 month follow-up, but differences between groups were small.*

- another study compared a group that wore cushioned shoe insoles *with* magnets to a group that wore cushioned shoe insoles *without* magnets (Winemiller 2003). *8 week follow-up showed that both groups improved, with no significant differences between them.* Other studies on magnetic shoe insoles have shown similar results (Caselli 1997).

- this study compared custom shoe inserts to over-the-counter arch supports to night splints (Martin 2001). *At 12 week follow-up, all groups improved with no significant differences between them.*

Taken as a whole, it appears that shoe inserts *are* effective in treating plantar fasciitis, with no differences between over-the-counter types and the more expensive custom-made inserts. As for magnets, don't waste your time.

night splints

As the name implies, these are splints you wear at night that look rather like big boots. The idea here is to try and keep foot and ankle structures stretched out all night in an effort to promote healing and avoid morning pain and stiffness that is so common in plantar fasciitis patients. Only a few randomized controlled trials have tested out this interesting idea:

- volunteers in one study were randomized to get either custom foot inserts, anterior night splints, or custom foot inserts *and* anterior night splints (Roos 2006). *At 12 weeks, all groups improved significantly with no significant differences found in pain among the three groups at any point in time.*

- in another study, patients wore either custom shoe inserts, over-the-counter arch supports, or night splints (Martin 2001). *At 12 week follow-up, all groups improved with no significant differences between them.*

- night splints were compared to no night splint use in this randomized controlled trial (Powell 1998). *After one month, the group that wore the night splints showed greater improvement compared to the control group.*

As you can see, night splints *are* effective in treating plantar fasciitis–but seem to be just as effective as over-the-counter or custom foot inserts! Given the choice between wearing a foot insert during the day or a plastic boot all night, well, let's just say it's your choice.

stretching the calf muscles

Calf muscle stretching, also known as Achilles tendon stretching, is designed to specifically stretch the calf muscles on the back of your lower leg, as well as that cable-like tendon in the back of your ankle, called the Achilles tendon. To my knowledge, there is only one randomized controlled trial that has tested the effectiveness of just doing calf muscle stretching alone in plantar fasciitis patients:

- in this study, one group of volunteers stretched their calf muscles for 3 minutes, three times daily, while another group did five 20-second stretches two times a day (Porter 2002). *At follow-up four months later, both groups improved with no differences in any aspect of their outcome.*

So it seems that based upon the *limited* evidence, calf muscle stretching *alone* is an effective treatment for plantar fasciitis. Note that the studies discussed in Chapter 3 that compare calf muscle stretching to plantar fascia stretching are not discussed here, because those studies had all participants also use shoe inserts and anti-inflammatory medications, and thus did not test the effects of just calf muscle stretching by itself.

extracorporeal shockwave therapy

Extracorporeal shockwave therapy, which is frequently used in the treatment of kidney stones, involves sending shock waves through the skin and into body tissues. Since the waves are created *outside* the body, they call it "extracorporeal" shockwave therapy. Proponents of using this treatment suggest that it does things such as stimulate soft tissue healing and inhibit pain impulse conduction–although the true effects have not been established and doses and regimes can widely vary. Here's what a compilation of the randomized, placebo-controlled, double-blinded (neither the patient nor the researcher knows who is getting which treatment) studies have to say of its effectiveness:

- volunteers in this study were randomized to receive either a single session of shockwave therapy or a placebo (fake) treatment (Kudo 2006). *6 week follow-up showed that the group that received the real shockwave therapy had significantly less pain.*

- in a similar study, participants were again randomized to receive either a single session of shockwave therapy or a placebo treatment session (Theodore 2004). *Three month follow-up showed 47% success in the placebo group compared to 56% success in the shockwave therapy group.*

- another study had participants receive either an active shockwave treatment or a fake one, monthly, for three months (Speed 2003). *Both groups showed significant improvement, with no significant differences existing between groups over a 6 month follow-up period.*

Looks like we have three, very well-done studies conducted in this area–two showing positive results and one negative. In a case like this, we clearly need more research to come to a solid conclusion, so until then, it's not unreasonable to give it a try as there is some support in the literature.

steroid injections

To my knowledge, there have been no randomized controlled trials evaluating steroid injections alone in the treatment of plantar fasciiits. Therefore, we do not know whether or not they are an effective treatment. Of interest, though, is this related randomized controlled trial:

- a 1998 study had plantar fasciitis sufferers receive either steroid injections/anti-inflammatory pills, **or** heel cup/pain pills, **or** taping/shoe inserts (Lynch 1998). *70% of the taping/shoe inserts group had an excellent or fair outcome compared to 33% of the group that received anti-inflammatory injections and medications.*

What's interesting here is that the group that received anti-inflammatory medication therapy, through injections and pills, did not do *nearly* as well as those who got their foot taped for four weeks while waiting for their custom shoe inserts (and then wore the inserts). This lends even more support to the notion that inflammation is not a key feature of plantar fasciitis–otherwise we would have expected the anti-inflammatory therapy to have had a much bigger impact than it did.

With there being no randomized controlled studies supporting the effectiveness of steroid injections alone, serious issues raised about inflammation being a part of plantar fasciitis, and the fact that there are *numerous* reports in the literature of plantar fascia *rupture* after one or more steroid injections (Acevedo 1998, Sellman 1994, Ahstrom 1988 and Leach 1978), it might be wise to be cautious with this particular treatment option.

surgery

Surgery done on plantar fasciitis patients to relieve symptoms involves cutting and releasing the fascia to varying degrees where it inserts at the heel. Here again, there are no randomized controlled trials that have been conducted to test out this treatment, so in all fairness, no one can really say one way or the other if it is truly effective or not. Remember, without a control group to compare things to, how do you know that someone who had their plantar fascia released and got better did well due to the surgery, or other factors such as the passing of time (i.e. Mother Nature)? The answer is, you don't know.

Readers should also be aware that cutting the plantar fascia can cause the arch of your foot to drop and flatten:

- a study done on cadavers (bodies donated to science) found that when the plantar fascia was completely cut and released, the foot arch dropped severly (Murphy 1998).

- another cadaver study calculated that after the plantar fascia was completely cut, arch stiffness decreased by twenty-five percent (Huang 1993).

- additionally, a 1997 cadaver study showed that even a *partial* release decreases the arch-supporting function of the plantar fascia in addition to weakening the structure (Thordarson 1997).

One could reasonably argue that those are all studies done on cadavers, and so the results may not be true in living patients. A good thought, but consider this study:

- 13 patients underwent plantar fasciotomy which entailed division of the central part of the plantar fascia (Daly 1992). Long-term follow-up, which ranged from a whopping 4.5 to 15 years, showed that patients had post-operative *flattening* of the foot arch.

Taking the above as a whole, *my advice* is that it would probably be best to consider this treatment option as a last resort because:

- there are no randomized controlled trials evaluating the effectiveness of surgery in treating plantar fasciitis

- cadaver studies, as well as long-term follow-up studies on actual patients show that releasing the plantar fascia causes the foot arch to drop which compromises foot stability

And that's it! As of this writing, those are all the treatments that have been tested out by themselves in randomized controlled trials (with the exception of the extracorporeal shockwave therapy where we looked at just the cream of the crop *double-blind* studies). While it is surprising that there aren't more, hopefully well-conducted future research will make this list significantly longer.

Summary

✓ if you want to know if a particular type of treatment is effective for a condition, the best thing to look for are randomized controlled trials that have tested it out by itself, without combining it with other treatments

✓ shoe inserts (custom or over-the-counter), night splints, calf muscle stretching and extracorporeal shockwave therapy have all been shown in randomized controlled trials to be effective as stand-alone treatments for plantar fasciitis

✓ magnetic shoe inserts, steroid injections, and surgery have not yet been demonstrated to be effective in treating plantar fasciitis in randomized controlled trials

Chapter Seven

Putting It All Together

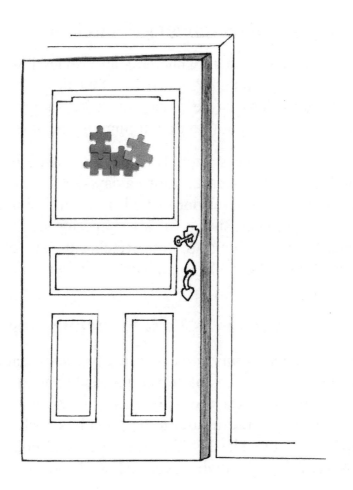

Putting It All Together

Well, we've come a long way since Chapter 1 and covered a lot of information. Unless you've been reading this book backwards, you should now have a good idea of what plantar fasciitis really is, how to get rid of it, and some things you can do to keep it from coming back. Having said that, it's time to begin the road to recovery. After getting the okay from your doctor, here's where to start...

Review the Stretching Technique and Begin

Begin by glancing back at Chapter 3 and reviewing the specific plantar fascia stretching technique. Practice it a few times, referring back to the pictures and instructions as necessary to make sure you're doing it right. After that, there's nothing left to do but jump in and start stretching.

Make sure you do the stretch 10 times in a row, holding for a *full* 10 seconds, and repeat this at least 3 times a day. *And above all*, make sure you do the stretch *before* you get out of bed in the morning and put weight on your foot. If you've been sitting for a long period of time without standing on your feet, the same thing applies–stretch out your plantar fascia *before* standing up. Remember, this timing is a *key* factor in helping the plantar fascia to finally heal.

Use the 8-Week Stretching Log

All the knowledge in this book is virtually *useless* unless you put in into action. So, I have two pieces of advice for readers who have trouble staying on track. The first is to use the daily exercise log, which you'll find on the next page. It is a very useful tool to help readers stick with their stretching and is easy to use–just check off a box when you complete one set of 10 stretches. Make a copy of it whenever you need another.

The second piece of advice? Check out, *"The Sixty-Second Motivator."* It too is a completely evidence-based book that I wrote specifically to help patients who have trouble motivating themselves to practice healthy habits such as exercising regularly or sticking to a healthy diet.

8-Week Stretching Log

Monday	Tuesday	Wednesday	Thursday	Friday	Saturday	Sunday
☐	☐	☐	☐	☐	☐	☐
☐	☐	☐	☐	☐	☐	☐
☐	☐	☐	☐	☐	☐	☐

Monday	Tuesday	Wednesday	Thursday	Friday	Saturday	Sunday
☐	☐	☐	☐	☐	☐	☐
☐	☐	☐	☐	☐	☐	☐
☐	☐	☐	☐	☐	☐	☐

Monday	Tuesday	Wednesday	Thursday	Friday	Saturday	Sunday
☐	☐	☐	☐	☐	☐	☐
☐	☐	☐	☐	☐	☐	☐
☐	☐	☐	☐	☐	☐	☐

Monday	Tuesday	Wednesday	Thursday	Friday	Saturday	Sunday
☐	☐	☐	☐	☐	☐	☐
☐	☐	☐	☐	☐	☐	☐
☐	☐	☐	☐	☐	☐	☐

Monday	Tuesday	Wednesday	Thursday	Friday	Saturday	Sunday
☐	☐	☐	☐	☐	☐	☐
☐	☐	☐	☐	☐	☐	☐
☐	☐	☐	☐	☐	☐	☐

Monday	Tuesday	Wednesday	Thursday	Friday	Saturday	Sunday
☐	☐	☐	☐	☐	☐	☐
☐	☐	☐	☐	☐	☐	☐
☐	☐	☐	☐	☐	☐	☐

Monday	Tuesday	Wednesday	Thursday	Friday	Saturday	Sunday
☐	☐	☐	☐	☐	☐	☐
☐	☐	☐	☐	☐	☐	☐
☐	☐	☐	☐	☐	☐	☐

Monday	Tuesday	Wednesday	Thursday	Friday	Saturday	Sunday
☐	☐	☐	☐	☐	☐	☐
☐	☐	☐	☐	☐	☐	☐
☐	☐	☐	☐	☐	☐	☐

Be Aware of Any Changes
In Pain *and* Function

As time passes, and you continue with the stretching, keep a sharp lookout for any changes in pain, those being:

- your foot pain is just as intense as always, however now it is occurring much less frequently

  or

- your foot pain is now *less* intense, even though it still occurring just as frequently

  or

- you start to notice less intense foot pain *and* it is now occurring less frequently

Additionally, make a copy of the Lower Extremity Functional Scale on page 40 and complete it every few weeks to monitor changes in your foot function. Remember, sometimes things *work* better before they begin to *feel* better. The bottom line? Any positive changes in pain or function you note indicates that the plantar fascia is finally beginning to heal.

Eliminate As Many Risk
Factors As You Can

Since there are no consistent reports in the scientific literature that plantar fasciitis has a high rate of recurrence, this part is optional. However, as they say, an ounce of prevention *is* worth a pound of cure, and anyone who's had plantar fasciitis is in no hurry to get it again.

Having said that, it might be worth your while to take a look at the three major risk factors discussed in Chapter 5—weighing too much, spending a lot of time on your feet, and not having a flexible ankle. Address any that may apply to you.

If All Else Fails, Try Plan "B"

Since the reality of the matter is that no one treatment will ever cure *everyone,* it's always good to have a plan "B". If you've tried the 5-Minute Plantar Fasciitis Solution diligently and consistently for a full 8-weeks, and have noticed not a lick of difference in pain or function, then it's time to check out some of the alternative treatments in Chapter 6. As always, discuss them with your doctor before trying any of them.

And that's it! Now that you have some good evidence-based knowledge and tools to work with, you stand a *very* good chance at beating one of the most common and annoying foot conditions to ever plague mankind. Good luck—I've enjoyed sharing my knowledge with you and hopefully you have found this a helpful and enlightening book.

-Jim Johnson, PT

Comprehensive List of Supporting References

Chapter 1

Akfirat M, et al.   Ultrasonographic appearance of the plantar fasciitis. *Journal of Clinical Imaging* 2003;27:353-357.

Berkowitz J, et al. Plantar fasciitis: MR imaging. *Radiology* 1991;179:665-667.

Cashmere T, et al.   Medial longitudinal arch of the foot: stationary versus walking measures. *Foot and Ankle International* 1999;20:112-118.

Genc H, et al. Long-term ultrasonographic follow-up of plantar fasciitis patients treated with steroid injection. *Joint Bone Spine* 2005;72:61-5.

Giacomozzi C, et al. Does the thickening of Achilles tendon and plantar fascia contribute to alteration of diabetic foot loading? *Clinical Biomechanics* 2005;20:532-539.

Gibbon W, et al. Ultrasound of the plantar aponeurosis (fascia). *Skeletal Radiol* 1999;28:21-26.

Huang C, et al. Biomechanical evaluation of longitudinal arch stability. *Foot and Ankle* 1993;14:353-357.

Hunt A, et al. Inter-segment foot motion and ground reaction forces over the stance phase of walking. *Clinical Biomechanics* 2001;16:592-600.

Hedrick M. The plantar aponeurosis. *Foot and Ankle International* 1996;17:646-649.

Hicks, J. The mechanics of the foot. II. The plantar aponeurosis and the arch. *J Anat* 1954;88:25-31.

Jarde O, et al. Degenerative lesions of the plantar fascia: surgical treatment by fasciectomy and excision of the heel spur. A report on 38 cases. *Acta Orthopaedica Belgica* 2003;69:267-274.

Kamel M, et al. High frequency ultrasonographic findings in plantar fasciitis and assessment of local steroid injection. *J Rheumatology* 2000;27:2139-2141.

Kane D, et al. The role of ultrasonography in the diagnosis and management of idiopathic plantar fasciitis. *Rheumatology* 2001;40:1002-1008.

Kappel-Bargas A, et al. The windlass mechanism during normal walking and passive first metatarsophalangeal joint extension. *Clinical Biomechanics* 1998;13:190-194.

Leach R, et al. Results of surgery in athletes with plantar fasciitis. *Foot and Ankle* 1986;7:156-161.

Lemont H, et al. Plantar fasciitis. A degenerative process (fasciosis) without inflammation. *Journal of the American Podiatric Medical Association* 2003;93:234-237.

Murphy G, et al. Biomechanical consequences of sequential plantar fascia release. *Foot and Ankle International* 1998;19:149-152.

Osborne HR, et al. Critical differences in lateral X-rays with and without a diagnosis of plantar fasciitis. *Journal of Science and Medicine in Sport* 2006;9:231-7.

Ozdemir H, et al. Sonographic evaluation of plantar fasciitis and relation to body mass index. *European Journal of Radiology* 2005;54:443-447.

Sabir N, et al. Clinical utility of sonography in diagnosing plantar fasciitis. *J Ultrasound Med* 2005;24:1041-1048.

Snider M, et al. Plantar fascia release for chronic plantar fasciitis in runners. *The American Journal of Sports Medicine* 1983;11:215-219.

Tountas A, et al. Operative treatment of subcalcaneal pain. Clinical Orthopaedics and Related Research 1996;332:170-178.

Uzel M, et al. The influence of athletic activity on the plantar fascia in healthy young adults. *Journal of Clinical Ultrasound* 2006;34:17-21.

Wall J, et al. Ultrasound diagnosis of plantar fasciitis. *Foot and Ankle* 1993;14:465-470.

Zhu F, et al. Chronic plantar fasciitis: Acute changes in the heel after extracorporeal high-energy shock wave therapy- observations at MR imaging. *Radiology* 2005;234:206-210.

Chapter 2

Davis P, et al. Painful heel syndrome: Results of nonoperative treatment. *Foot and Ankle International* 1994;15:531-535.

Landorf K, et al. Effectiveness of foot orthoses to treat plantar fasciitis. *Archives of Internal Medicine* 2006;166:1305-1310.

Radford J, et al. Effectiveness of low-dye taping for the short-term treatment of plantar heel pain: a randomized trial. *BMC Musculoskeletal Disorders* 2006;7:64-70.

Speed C, et al. Extracorporeal shock wave therapy for plantar fasciitis. A double blind randomised controlled trial. *Journal of Orthopaedic Research* 2003;21:937-940.

Wolgin M, et al. Conservative treatment of plantar heel pain: Long-term follow-up. *Foot and Ankle* 1994;15;97-102.

Chapter 3

DiGiovanni B, et al. Tissue-specific plantar fascia-stretching exercise enhances outcomes in patients with chronic heel pain. *Journal of Bone and Joint Surgery* 2003;85-A;1270-1277.

DiGiovanni B, et al. Plantar fascia-specific stretching exercise improves outcomes in patients with chronic plantar fasciitis. *Journal of Bone and Joint Surgery* 2006;88-A;1775-1781.

Chapter 4

Binkley J, et al. The lower extremity functional scale (LEFS): Scale development, measurement properties, and clinical application. *Physical Therapy* 1999;79:371-383.

Martin, R, et al. A survey of self-reported outcome instruments for the foot and ankle. *Journal of Orthopaedic and Sports Physical Therapy* 2007;37:72-84.

Riddle D, et al. Impact of demographic and impairment-related variables on disability associated plantar fasciitis. *Foot and Ankle International* 2004;25:311-317.

Chapter 5

Akfirat M, et al. Ultrasonographic appearance of the plantar fasciitis. *Journal of Clinical Imaging* 2003;27:353-357.

Allen R, et al. Toe flexors strength and passive extension range of motion of the first metatarsophalangeal joint in individuals with plantar fasciitis. *Journal of Orthopaedic and Sports Physical Therapy* 2003;33:468-478.

Berkowitz J, et al. Plantar fasciitis: MR imaging. *Radiology* 1991;179:665-667.

Bohannon R, et al. Effect of five minute stretch on ankle dorsiflexion range of motion. *J Phys Ther Sci* 1994;6:1-8.

Creighton D, et al. Evaluation of range of motion of the first metatarsophalangeal joint in runners with plantar fasciitis. *Journal of Orthopaedic and Sports Physical Therapy 1987;8:357-361.*

Forman W, et al. The role of intrinsic musculature in the formation of inferior calcaneal exostoses. *Clinics in Podiatric Medicine and Surgery* 1990;7:217-223.

Knight C, et al. Effect of superficial heat, deep heat, and active exercise warm-up on the extensibility of the plantar flexors. *Physical Therapy* 2001;81:1206-1214.

Gajdosik R, et al. A stretching program increases the dynamic passive length and passive resistive properties of the calf muscle-tendon unit of unconditioned younger women. *Eur J Appl Physiol* 2007;99:449-454.

Gajdosik R, et al. Effects of an eight-week stretching program on the passive-elastic properties and function of the calf muscles of older women. *Clinical Biomechanics* 2005;20:973-983.

McCarthy D, et al. The anatomical basis of inferior calcaneal lesions. *Journal of the American Podiatry Association* 1979;69:527-536.

Osborne HR, et al. Critical differences in lateral X-rays with and without a diagnosis of plantar fasciitis. *Journal of Science and Medicine in Sport* 2006;9:231-7.

Peres S, et al. Pulsed shortwave diathermy and prolonged long-duration stretching increase dorsiflexion range of motion more than identical stretching without diathermy. *Journal of Athletic Training* 2002;37:43-50.

Pratt K, et al. Effects of a 3-minute standing stretch on ankle-dorsiflexion range of motion, *J Sport Rehabil* 2003;12:162-173.

Prichasuk S. The heel pad in plantar heel pain. *Journal of Bone and Joint Surgery* 1994;76-B:140-2.

Prichasuk S, et al. The relationship of pes planus and calcaneal spur to plantar heel pain. *Clinical Orthopaedics and Related Research* 1994;306:192-196.

Riddle D, et al. Risk factors for plantar fasciitis: A matched case-control study. *Journal of Bone and Joint Surgery* 2003;85-A:872-877.

Wearing S, et al. Sagittal movement of the medial longitudinal arch is unchanged in plantar fasciitis. *Medicine and Science in Sports and Exercise* 2004;36:1761-1767.

Youdas J, et al. The effect of static stretching of the calf muscle-tendon unit on active ankle dorsiflexion range of motion. *Journal of Orthopaedic and Sports Physical Therapy* 2003;33:408-417.

Chapter 6

Acevedo J, et al. Complications of plantar fascia rupture associated with corticosteroid injection. *Foot and Ankle International* 1998;19:91-97.

Ahstrom J. Spontaneous rupture of the plantar fascia. *The American Journal of Sports Medicine* 1988;16:306-307.

Caselli M, et al. Evaluation of magnetic foil and PPT insoles in the treatment of heel pain. *Journal of the American Podiatric Medical Association* 1997;87:11-16.

Daly P, et al. Plantar fasciotomy for intractable plantar fasciitis: Clinical results and biomechanical evaluation. *Foot and Ankle* 1992;13:188-195.

Huang C, et al. Biomechanical evaluation of longitudinal arch stability. *Foot and Ankle* 1993;14:353-357.

Kudo P, et al. Randomized, placebo-controlled, double-blind clinical trial evaluating the treatment of plantar fasciitis with an extracorporeal shockwave therapy (ESWT) device: A North American confirmatory study. *Journal of Orthopaedic Research* 2006:24:115-123.

Landorf K, et al. Effectiveness of foot orthoses to treat plantar fasciitis. *Archives of Internal Medicine* 2006;166:1305-1310.

Leach R, et al. Rupture of the plantar fascia in athletes. *The Journal of Bone and Joint Surgery* 1978;60-A:537-539.

Lynch D, et al. Conservative treatment of plantar fasciitis. A prospective study. *Journal of the American Podiatric Medical Association* 1998;88:375-380.

Murphy G, et al. Biomechanical consequences of sequential plantar fascia release. *Foot and Ankle International* 1998;19:149-152.

Martin J, et al. Mechanical treatment of plantar fasciitis. A prospective study. *Journal of the American Podiatric Medical Association* 2001;91:55-62.

Porter D, et al. The effects of duration and frequency of Achilles tendon stretching on dorsiflexion and outcome in painful heel syndrome: A randomized, blinded, control study. *Foot and Ankle International* 2002;23:619-624.

Powell M, et al. Effective treatment of chronic plantar fasciitis with dorsiflexion night splints: A crossover prospective randomized outcome study. *Foot and Ankle International* 1998;19:10-18.

Roos E, et al. Foot orthoses for the treatment of plantar fasciitis. *Foot and Ankle International* 2006;27:606-611.

Sellman J. Plantar fascia rupture associated with corticosteroid injection. *Foot and Ankle International* 1994;15:376-381.

Speed C, et al. Extracorporeal shock wave therapy for plantar fasciitis. A double blind randomised controlled trial. *Journal of Orthopaedic Research* 2003;21:937-940.

Theodore G, et al. Extracorporeal shock wave therapy for the treatment of plantar fasciitis. *Foot and Ankle International* 2004;25:290-297.

Thordarson D, et al. Effect of partial versus complete plantar fasciotomy on the windlass mechanism. *Foot and Ankle International* 1997;18:16-20.

Winemiller M, et al. Effect of magnetic vs sham-magnetic insoles on plantar heel pain. A randomized controlled trial. *JAMA* 2003;290:1474-1478.

Lightning Source UK Ltd.
Milton Keynes UK
29 December 2010

164962UK00004B/7/P